Table of Contents

PREVIEW

Narcolepsy is a chronic sleep disorder characterized by overwhelming daytime drowsiness and sudden attacks of sleep. People with narcolepsy often find it difficult to stay awake for long periods of time, regardless of the circumstances. Narcolepsy can cause serious disruptions in your daily routine.

Sometimes, narcolepsy can be accompanied by a sudden loss of muscle tone (cataplexy), which can be triggered by strong emotion. Narcolepsy that occurs with cataplexy is called type 1 narcolepsy. Narcolepsy that occurs without cataplexy is known as type 2 narcolepsy.

Narcolepsy is a chronic condition for which there's no cure. However, medications and lifestyle changes can help you manage the symptoms. Support from others — family, friends, employers, teachers — can help you cope with narcolepsy.

NARCOLEPSY DIET RECIPES

BREAKFAST

1. Copycat Starbucks Egg Bites

Prep Time: 10-15 mins

Cook Time: 18-22 mins

Total Time: 28-37 mins

Yield: Makes 12 bites

Ingredients

- 1 teaspoon olive oil
- ½ medium red bell pepper, seeded and diced
- 2 cups fresh baby spinach, chopped (optional)
- 8 large eggs
- ½ cup plain Greek yogurt, cottage cheese or ricotta
- 1 ½ teaspoons coarse salt
- 1 teaspoon onion powder
- 1 teaspoon garlic powder
- 1 teaspoon mustard powder
- ½ teaspoon ground black pepper

- ½ cup diced ham
- ¼ cup shredded Gruyere or white cheddar

Instructions

1. Preheat the oven to 350 degrees.

2. Heat olive oil in a large skillet to medium. Add the bell pepper and spinach (if using) and sauté 2-3 minutes or until the peppers are slightly soft. Set aside.

3. Place the eggs, Greek yogurt, cottage cheese or ricotta, salt, onion powder, garlic powder, mustard powder and black pepper in a blender. Puree until smooth.

4. Coat a 12-cup muffin tin with cooking spray. Pour the egg mixture into each of the muffin cups, filling about ¾ of the way to the top.

5. Spoon a small spoonful of the pepper mixture and the diced ham into each cup. Top each with shredded Gruyere or white cheddar.

6. Bake 18-22 minutes or until egg is set. Let slightly cool, then run a knife around the edge of each muffin

and carefully remove from the muffin tin cup. Serve immediately or let cool and store in airtight containers in the refrigerator up to 5 days or the freezer up to 2 months.

Prep Time: 5 min

Cook Time: 10 min

Total Time: 15 min

Yield: Serves 6

Ingredients

- 3 ½–4 cups water
- 1 ½ cups old-fashioned rolled oats
- ½ cup chia seeds
- ½ tablespoon ground cinnamon
- 1 teaspoon pure vanilla extract
- ½ teaspoon coarse salt
- ½ cup natural peanut butter
- ½ cup milk of choice + more for serving
- 3 tablespoons pure maple syrup + more for serving
- 2 tablespoons butter
- 1 teaspoon brown sugar
- 3 yellow bananas, peeled and sliced
- ½ cup chopped walnuts and/or sliced almonds

Instructions

1. Bring water to a boil in a large saucepan. Pour oats and chia seeds into the water, bring to a boil, then reduce to a simmer for about 5 minutes, stirring frequently, until oats are soft. Remove from heat and stir in cinnamon, vanilla extract, salt, peanut butter, milk and maple syrup until combined.

2. In a medium skillet, melt butter and brown sugar at medium-high heat. Add sliced bananas and cook 1-2 minutes per side, until browned, flipping once.

3. Scoop oatmeal into bowls and top with milk and maple syrup, as desired, and walnuts/almonds and caramelized bananas.

Prep Time: 10 mins

Cook Time: 12 mins

Total Time: 22 mins

Yield: 18 cookies

Ingredients

Cookies:

- 2 cups old-fashioned rolled oats
- 1 cup whole wheat pastry flour (or whole wheat flour)
- ½ teaspoon baking soda
- ½ teaspoon coarse salt
- ½ teaspoon ground cinnamon
- ⅓ cup oil
- ½ cup brown sugar
- 2 large eggs
- ⅔ cup vanilla yogurt
- 2 teaspoons pure vanilla extract

Mix-Ins:

- 2–3 tablespoons dark chocolate chips + 2–3 tablespoons unsweetened coconut flakes

- ½ small banana, smashed + ¼ cup blueberries
- 2 tablespoons peanut butter + 2 tablespoons strawberry preserves

Instructions

1. Preheat oven to 350 degrees. Line a large baking sheet with parchment paper.

2. In a medium mixing bowl, whisk together oats, flour, baking soda, salt and cinnamon.

3. In another medium mixing bowl, whisk together oil and brown sugar, until fluffy. Whisk in eggs, until incorporated, then whisk in vanilla yogurt and vanilla extract. Pour dry ingredients into wet ingredients and whisk until just combined.

4. Fold in desired mix-ins. Scoop dough using a 2-inch cookie scoop, about 1-inch apart on the baking sheet. Bake 9-12 minutes. Allow to slightly cool.

Prep Time: 10-15 mins

Cook Time: 20-25 mins

Total Time: 30-40 mins

Yield: Makes 12 muffins

Ingredients

Topping:

- 4 tablespoons butter
- ½ cup old-fashioned rolled oats
- 2 tablespoons brown sugar
- 1 teaspoon cinnamon

Muffins:

- 2 large ripe bananas
- ½ cup brown sugar
- 2 large eggs
- ¼ cup oil
- 1 cup oat flour (or ground oats)
- ½ + ⅔ cup rolled old-fashioned oats
- 1 teaspoon baking powder
- 1 teaspoon baking soda

- ½ teaspoon coarse salt
- ½ cup dark chocolate chips or fresh or frozen blueberries (if using)

Instructions

1. Preheat oven to 350 degrees. Coat an 8 or 12-cup muffin tin with cooking spray.

2. In a small bowl, melt the butter. Add oats, brown sugar and cinnamon and stir to combine. Set aside.

3. In the bowl of a stand mixer, cream bananas, brown sugar, eggs and oil until fluffy. In a separate medium bowl, whisk together oat flour, oats, baking powder, baking soda and salt. While the mixer is running, slowly dump dry ingredients into the banana mixture, just until combined. Fold in chocolate chips or blueberries (if using). Spoon batter into muffin tin, about ⅔ of the way full. Top each muffin with a spoonful of topping. Bake 18-22 minutes, until toothpick inserted into the center of a muffin comes out clean. Allow to cool.

Prep Time: 10 mins

Cook Time: 25 mins

Total Time: 35 mins

Yield: 20 Cups

Ingredients

- 8 large eggs
- 2 ½ cups milk
- ¼ cup + 2 tablespoons pure maple syrup, divided
- 1 ½ tablespoons ground cinnamon
- 2 teaspoons pure vanilla extract
- 1 teaspoon almond extract (optional)
- ¼ teaspoon coarse salt
- Pinch ground cloves
- 1 loaf whole grain cinnamon bread, cubed
- 2 cups fresh or frozen whole cranberries

Instructions

1. Preheat oven to 375 degrees. Coat two 12-cup muffin tins with cooking spray. Set aside.

2. In an extra-large mixing bowl, whisk together eggs, milk, ¼ cup maple syrup, cinnamon, vanilla extract, almond extract (if using), salt and ground cloves. Stir in cubed bread and cranberries until thoroughly combined.

3. Scoop mixture into muffin tin cups to the brim. Drizzle with remaining maple syrup. Bake 20-25 minutes, until set and browned on top. Let slightly cool before removing from muffin tins.

Prep Time: 10 mins

Cook Time: 20 mins

Total Time: 30 mins

Yield: 9 Muffins

Ingredients

Topping:

- ¼ cup rolled old-fashioned oats
- ¼ cup slivered almonds
- ¼ cup butter, melted
- 2 tablespoons brown sugar
- 1 teaspoon ground cinnamon

Muffins:

- ¾ cup brown sugar
- 2 large eggs
- 6 tablespoons oil
- ¼ cup milk
- 2 teaspoons vanilla extract
- 1 ½ cups whole wheat pastry or oat flour*
- ½ cup rolled old-fashioned oats

- 1 ½ teaspoons baking powder
- 1 teaspoon baking soda
- ½ teaspoon coarse salt
- ½ teaspoon ground ginger
- 1 cup fresh or frozen cranberries

Instructions

1. Preheat oven to 350 degrees.

2. In a small bowl, combine the topping ingredients. Set aside.

3. In a medium mixing bowl, whisk together brown sugar, eggs, oil, milk and vanilla extract until combined.

4. In another medium mixing bowl, whisk together oat flour, oats, baking powder, baking soda, salt and ginger. Pour dry ingredients into the bowl of wet ingredients and whisk together until just combined. Fold in cranberries.

5. Spoon batter into the wells of a greased 9-cup muffin tin, about ¾ of the way full. Top with a scoop of the oat/almond topping. Bake 18-20 minutes, until

toothpick inserted into the center of the muffin comes out clean. Allow to cool.

Prep Time: 10-15 mins

Cook Time: 20-25 mins

Total Time: 30-40 mins

Yield: Serves 8

Ingredients

- 10 large eggs
- ½ cup Greek yogurt
- 1 ½ teaspoons coarse salt
- 1 teaspoon dried oregano leaves
- 1 teaspoon chili powder
- 1 teaspoon onion powder
- ½ teaspoon garlic powder
- ½ teaspoon ground black pepper
- 4 ounces ground chorizo
- 3 cups fresh baby spinach
- 2 cups steamed cauliflower florets
- ½ cup shredded pepperjack cheese
- ¼ cup fresh cilantro, chopped

Instructions

1. Preheat oven to 350 degrees.

2. In a large bowl, whisk together the eggs, Greek yogurt, salt, oregano, chili powder, onion powder, garlic and black pepper until thoroughly combined. Set aside.

3. Heat a large nonstick oven-safe skillet or stove top casserole dish to medium. Add the chorizo and cook 2-3 minutes, breaking up with a spatula, until browned. Stir in the spinach and cook 1-2 minutes or until wilted. Reduce the heat to medium-low.

4. Push the chorizo and spinach mixture aside in the skillet or casserole dish to coat with cooking spray. Add the egg mixture to the pan and gently stir to incorporate the chorizo and spinach. Evenly distribute the cauliflower florets among the egg mixture. Top with the pepperjack cheese and cilantro. Once the sides start to bubble up and cook, remove from the stove and place in the oven. Cook 15-20 minutes or until set. Let slightly cool, then slice into wedges and serve.

8. Lemon Ricotta Pancakes

Prep Time: 10-15 mins

Cook Time: 10-15 mins

Total Time: 20-30 mins

Yield: Serves 5

Ingredients

Berry Compote:

- 1 ½ cups fresh or frozen blueberries
- Zest and juice of ½ medium lemon (about 1 tablespoon)
- ½ tablespoon granulated sugar

Lemon Ricotta Pancakes:

- 1 ¼ cups whole wheat or oat flour
- 1 tablespoon granulated sugar
- 2 teaspoons baking powder
- ½ teaspoon baking soda
- ¼ teaspoon kosher or sea salt
- 1 cup ricotta cheese
- 2 large eggs, yolks and white separated
- Zest and juice of 2 medium lemons (about ¼ cup)

- ¼ cup milk

- 2 tablespoons oil

- 1 teaspoon pure vanilla extract

Instructions

1. Stir together the blueberries, lemon zest and juice, and sugar in a small saucepan. Bring to a low simmer for 10-15 minutes, stirring occasionally, until slightly thickened. Remove from the heat and set aside.

2. In a large mixing bowl, stir together the flour, sugar, baking powder, baking soda, and salt.

3. In a separate medium mixing bowl, whisk together ricotta cheese and egg yolks until fluffy. Whisk in the lemon zest and juice, milk, oil, and vanilla extract until combined. Fold in the dry ingredients until combined.

4. Place the egg whites in a separate bowl. Use a hand mixer to whip the egg whites until stiff peaks form. Gently fold the egg whites into the batter, just until combined.

5. Heat a large skillet to medium-high heat. Coat with cooking spray. Working in batches, pour ¼ cup batter into the hot skillet and cook 2-3 minutes per side, until set. Repeat with remaining batter.

6. Serve the pancakes with blueberry compote.

Prep Time: 15 mins

Cook Time: 40-45 mins

Total Time: 55-60 mins

Yield: Serves 16

Ingredients

- ¾ cup granulated sugar
- ⅔ cup softened butter and/or oil
- 2 large eggs
- 1 tablespoon vanilla extract
- 1 ½ cups all-purpose flour
- 1 ½ cups whole wheat or whole wheat pastry flour
- 4 teaspoons baking powder
- ½ teaspoon salt
- 1 ½ cups plain Greek yogurt or milk
- ⅓ cup packed dark brown sugar
- 4 teaspoons ground cinnamon

Instructions

1. Preheat the oven to 375 degrees. Line an 8-inch square baking dish with parchment paper.

2. In a mixing bowl, cream together granulated sugar, butter and/or oil, egg and vanilla extract.

3. In a separate bowl, combine all-purpose flour, whole wheat flour, baking powder and salt.

4. Add flour mixture to sugar mixture alternately with milk or yogurt, mixing after each addition. Spread half of the batter into the prepared pan.

5. In a small bowl or measuring cup, mix brown sugar and cinnamon and sprinkle half over the batter. Add remaining batter and carefully spread over cinnamon sugar mixture. Top batter with remaining cinnamon sugar mixture.

6. Bake 40-45 minutes or until a wooden pick inserted in the center comes out clean.

Prep Time: 15 min

Cook Time: 0 min

Total Time: 15 min + 4 hrs refrigeration

Yield: Serves 4

Ingredients

Chocolate Overnight Oats:

- 1 ½ cups old-fashioned rolled oats
- 2 ¼ cups milk*
- 3 tablespoons maple syrup or honey
- 2 tablespoons unsweetened cocoa powder
- Pinch coarse salt

Raspberry Chia Pudding:

- ½ cup chia seeds
- 2 ½ cups milk*
- 2 tablespoons maple syrup or honey
- 1 teaspoon pure vanilla extract
- 1 cup raspberries

Parfaits:

- 1 cup raspberries
- ¼ cup mini dark chocolate chips (optional)

Instructions

1. In a medium bowl, thoroughly whisk together the oats, milk, maple syrup or honey, cocoa powder and a pinch of salt. Set aside for 5 minutes, then whisk again. Cover and refrigerate for at least 4 hours.

2. In another medium bowl, thoroughly whisk together chia seeds, milk, maple syrup or honey, vanilla extract and salt. Add the raspberries and use the back of a fork to mash them. Stir to combine. Set aside for 5 minutes, then whisk again. Cover and refrigerate for at least 4 hours.

3. Prepare parfaits by laying the overnight oats and chia pudding in 4 medium jars. Top with raspberries and mini dark chocolate chips (if using). Cover and store up to 4 days.

11. Salmon Nicoise Salad

Prep Time: 10-15 mins

Cook Time: 6-10 mins

Total Time: 16-25 mins

Yield: Serves 6

Ingredients

Lemon Dressing:

- Zest and juice of 2 medium lemons
- 1 tablespoon Dijon mustard
- ½ tablespoon honey
- ⅓ cup olive oil
- ½ teaspoon coarse salt
- ¼ teaspoon ground black pepper

Niçoise Salad:

- ½ pound baby Yukon or red potatoes, halved
- 1-pound green beans, trimmed
- 6 cups butter lettuce
- 6 hard-boiled or soft-boiled eggs, halved

- 4 mini cucumbers or 1 medium English cucumber, sliced
- 1-pint cherry or grape tomatoes, halved
- ½ cup Greek or kalamata olives

Salmon:

- 1 tablespoon olive oil
- 1-pound fresh salmon, skin removed
- ½ teaspoon coarse salt
- ¼ teaspoon ground black pepper

Instructions

1. Bring a large pot of salted water to a boil.

2. In a small bowl, whisk together the lemon zest and juice, Dijon mustard, honey, olive oil, salt and black pepper. Taste and adjust seasoning, if necessary. Refrigerate until ready to use.

3. Add the potatoes to the boiling water and cook 5 minutes. Add the green beans and cook the potatoes and beans another 3-4 minutes. Transfer to a large bowl of ice water. Use a slotted spoon to transfer the

potatoes and green beans to a paper towel-lined plate to dry.

4. Arrange salad bowls with butter lettuce, potatoes, green beans, eggs, cucumbers, tomatoes and olives. Set aside.

5. Heat the olive oil in a large nonstick skillet or cast-iron pan to medium heat. Season the salmon with salt and black pepper. Once the pan is hot, add the salmon and cook 2-3 minutes per side or until it just starts to flake when gently pressed with the back of a fork. Let slightly cool, then transfer salmon pieces to the salad bowls.

6. Drizzle lemon dressing on each salad and serve immediately.

Prep Time: 15 min

Cook Time: 0 min

Total Time: 15 min

Yield: Serves 4

Ingredients

Vinaigrette:

- 3 tablespoons balsamic vinegar
- 2 tablespoons honey
- 1 tablespoon Dijon mustard
- ¼ cup olive oil
- ¼ teaspoon coarse salt
- ¼ teaspoon freshly ground black pepper

Salad:

- 4–6 cups spring mix
- 4 (4- to 6-ounce) cooked boneless skinless chicken breasts, cooled and sliced

- 2–3 cups fresh berries (strawberries, blackberries, blueberries)

- 1 medium ripe avocado, peeled and sliced

- ½ cup cooked quinoa, cooled

- Pinch of coarse salt and freshly ground black pepper, if desired

- Handful chopped walnuts or almonds and feta, goat or Parmesan cheese, if desired

Instructions

1. In a small measuring cup or bowl, whisk together dressing ingredients. Taste and adjust seasoning, if necessary.

2. Arrange spring mix in bowls. Distribute chicken breasts, berries, avocado and quinoa on each salad. Sprinkle lightly with salt and freshly ground black pepper, if desired. Top with nuts and cheese, if desired.

3. Just before serving, drizzle dressing on salad. Store leftover salad and dressing in separate containers in the refrigerator.

Prep Time: 15 mins

Cook Time: 0 mins

Total Time: 15 mins

Yield: Serves 4

Ingredients

Feta Vinaigrette

- Zest and juice of 1 medium lemon (about ¼ cup)
- 2 tablespoons red wine vinegar
- 2 cloves garlic, peeled and minced
- 1 tablespoon granulated sugar + 1 tsp. honey
- 1 teaspoon dried oregano leaves
- ½ teaspoon dried basil leaves
- ½ cup extra virgin olive oil
- Dash coarse salt and ground black pepper
- ¼ cup crumbled feta cheese

Greek Salad

- 3 heads romaine lettuce, chopped
- 1 English cucumber, halved and thinly sliced
- 1 green bell pepper, thinly sliced

- ½ pint cherry tomatoes
- ½ cup pitted kalamata olives
- ½ cup crumbled feta cheese
- Dash coarse salt and ground black pepper
- ¼ cup shaved Parmesan cheese
- Whole pepperoncini, for garnish (optional)

Instructions

1. Whisk together lemon zest and juice, vinegar, garlic, sugar, honey, oregano and basil. Drizzle in olive oil until combined. Season with salt and black pepper and taste; adjust seasoning if necessary. Whisk in feta cheese. Set aside.

2. In a large bowl, combine romaine lettuce, cucumber, bell pepper, tomatoes, olives and feta cheese. Toss with desired amount of dressing. Sprinkle with coarse salt and black pepper and top with Parmesan cheese and garnish with pepperoncini, if desired.

Prep Time: 20 min

Cook Time: 30 min

Total Time: 50 min

Yield: Serves 10

Ingredients

- 6 large eggs
- 2 ½–3 lbs. baby Yukon gold potatoes, halved or quartered
- ½ cup olive oil
- 3 tablespoons Dijon mustard
- 2 tablespoons white wine vinegar
- 1 tablespoon honey
- ¾–1 teaspoon coarse salt
- ½ teaspoon ground black pepper
- 3–4 stalks celery, diced and/or 3–4 scallions, sliced
- Handful of freshly chopped herbs, for garnish

Instructions

1. Place eggs in a medium saucepan and cover with cold water. Place over high heat and bring to a boil. Once

the water boils, shut the heat off and place a lid on the pan. Set a timer for 16-17 minutes. When the timer goes off, drain water and either rinse eggs with cold water or place in an ice water bath until chilled. Peel and discard shells. Chop eggs into quarters.

2. Bring a large pot of water to a boil. Add potatoes and simmer until just tender, about 10-12 minutes. Drain and rinse with cold water.

3. In a large mixing bowl, whisk together olive oil, Dijon, vinegar, honey, salt and black pepper. Taste and adjust seasoning, if necessary. Fold in potatoes, eggs and celery/scallions until combined. Place a lid on the bowl and refrigerate until chilled.

4. Transfer to a serving bowl and garnish with chopped fresh herbs.

15. Chocolate-Dipped Peanut Butter Cereal Bars

Prep Time: 15 mins

Cook Time: 5 mins

Total Time: 20 mins

Yield: Makes 18 bars

Ingredients

- ½ cup creamy peanut butter
- ¼ cup + 1 tablespoon coconut oil
- 3 tablespoons pure maple syrup
- 2 tablespoons honey
- 1 ½ teaspoons pure vanilla extract
- ¼ teaspoon coarse salt
- 3 cups multi-grain Cheerios
- ⅓ cup dark chocolate chips

Instructions

1. Line a large sheet of parchment paper in an 8×8 baking dish. Set aside.

2. Place the peanut butter, coconut oil, maple syrup and honey in a large microwaveable bowl. Microwave on high in 30 second increments, stirring in between,

until coconut oil is melted, about 1 minute 30 seconds to 2 minutes total. Add the vanilla extract and salt and stir to thoroughly combine.

3. Add the Cheerios and stir to combine. Transfer to the prepared baking dish and press until mixture is evenly distributed and flat. Refrigerate at least 30 minute or until set. Grab the edges of the parchment paper and transfer the bars to a cutting board. Cut into 18 small squares.

4. Place the chocolate chips in a small microwaveable bowl. Microwave on high in 30 second increments, stirring in between, until chocolate is melted, about 1 minute 30 seconds. Dip the bottom of each bar in the chocolate and transfer back to the parchment paper. Let sit until hardened, about 30 minutes.

5. Store in an airtight container in the refrigerator for up to a week.

16. White Chocolate Peppermint Brownie Cookies

Prep Time: 10 min

Cook Time: 15 min

Total Time: 25 min

Yield: Makes 12 cookies

Ingredients

- 1 ½ cups dark chocolate chips
- 2 tablespoons butter
- 2 large eggs
- ¾ cup granulated sugar
- ½ teaspoon pure vanilla extract
- ¼ cup all-purpose flour
- ¼ teaspoon baking powder
- ½ cup chopped white chocolate peppermint bars

Instructions

1. Place chocolate chips and butter in a glass bowl. Microwave in 30 second increments, stirring in between each, until melted.

2. In a separate bowl, use a hand mixer to whip eggs until fluffy. Add sugar and continue to beat until

fluffy and pale-colored. Beat in vanilla extract. Slowly beat in chocolate mixture until combined. Sift in flour and baking powder and fold until just combined. Fold in chopped white chocolate peppermint pieces. Cover the bowl and refrigerate 1 hour.

3. Preheat the oven to 350 degrees. Line baking sheets with parchment paper. Use a medium cookie scoop to form balls of dough. Line 2-inches apart on the cookie sheets. Gently press each until slightly flattened. Bake 10-15 minutes.

Prep Time: 30 min

Cook Time: 50 min

Total Time: 1 hr 20 mins

Yield: Serves 8

Ingredients

Pie Crust:

- 1 3/4 cups all-purpose flour + more for dusting
- ¼ teaspoon coarse salt
- 8 tablespoons (1 stick) cold butter, cubed
- 4–6 tablespoons ice water

Pie Filling:

- 3/4 cup dark brown sugar
- 1 ½ teaspoon ground cinnamon
- ¾ teaspoon ground ginger
- ½ teaspoon coarse salt
- ¼ teaspoon ground nutmeg
- ¼ teaspoon ground cloves
- 2 large eggs
- 2 ½ cups mashed sweet potatoes

- 1 (12-ounce) can evaporated milk

- 2 teaspoons pure vanilla extract

- 2 tablespoons turbinado sugar (optional)

Whipped Cream:

- 1 cup heavy whipping cream

- 3 tablespoons pure maple syrup

- 1 teaspoon pure vanilla extract

Instructions

1. Whisk together flour and salt in a large mixing bowl. Add cubed butter and use a pastry cutter to cut the butter into the flour until pea-sized granules form. Add ice water, 1 tablespoon at a time, until it resembles wet sand. Transfer the mixture onto a floured cutting board and work into a ball. Wrap in plastic wrap and place in the refrigerator for 30 minutes.

2. In a large mixing bowl, stir together brown sugar, cinnamon, ginger, salt, nutmeg and cloves. Use a hand mixer to beat in eggs, one at a time, until fluffy. Beat in sweet potatoes until smooth. Slowly

beat in evaporated milk and vanilla extract. Set aside.

3. Preheat oven to 425 degrees.

4. Remove cold dough from the plastic wrap and place on the floured cutting board. Use a rolling pin to roll it into a 1/4 inch thick round. Place into a deep-dish pie plate. Trim the edges into a perfect circle, hanging over about 1/4 inch. Fold the edges under and pinch the edges using your thumbs.

5. Pour the sweet potato mixture into the crust. Bake at 425 degrees for 15 minutes, then reduce the heat to 350 and bake an additional 30-35 minutes or until pie is no longer jiggly and crust is lightly browned. Let completely cool.

6. Optional: Sprinkle turbinado sugar in one even layer on the pie. Use a kitchen torch to 'brulee' the sugar until a crisp crust forms, being careful not to burn the sugar or pie crust. Let cool, then cut into slices.

7. In the bowl of a stand mixer, whip heavy cream on high speed. Drizzle in maple syrup and vanilla and continue to whip until stiff peaks form. Dollop whipped cream on each slice of pie and serve.

18. Pumpkin Chocolate Chip Mini Scones

Prep Time: 20 min

Cook Time: 15 min

Total Time: 35 min

Yield: 16 scones

Ingredients

Scones:

- 2 cups all-purpose flour + ~¼ cup for dusting
- 1 ½ cups whole wheat pastry flour
- 1 tablespoon baking powder
- ½ tablespoon pumpkin pie spice
- ½ teaspoon coarse salt
- 6 tablespoons cold salted butter, cut into cubes
- 2 large eggs
- ¾ cup dark brown sugar
- 1 cup pumpkin puree
- 1 teaspoon pure vanilla extract
- 1 cup dark chocolate chips

Glaze:

- ½ cup powdered sugar

- 1 tablespoon milk

- 1 tablespoon pure maple syrup

- ¼ cup pepitas (pumpkin seeds), crushed

Instructions

1. Preheat the oven to 375 degrees. Line a baking sheet with parchment paper and set aside.

2. In the bowl of a stand mixer, whisk together flours, baking powder, pie spice and salt. Add cold butter cubes and run mixer on low, incorporating the butter until it forms pea-sized rounds.

3. In a separate medium bowl, whisk together eggs, brown sugar, pumpkin and vanilla extract. Slowly pour wet ingredients into the stand mixer on low until a wet dough forms. Add chocolate chips and mix for 10-15 seconds. Do not overmix.

4. Place dough on a floured cutting board. Work with your hands to form a ball. Divide dough into two balls. Flatten into a round shape, about 1 inch thick. Wrap with plastic wrap and refrigerate about 30 minutes. Place back on the cutting board and cut each

dough round into 8 mini triangles. Transfer to the parchment paper.

5. Bake 13-16 minutes until lightly browned and fluffy. Remove and cool. In a small bowl, whisk together powdered sugar, milk and maple extract or syrup until glaze forms. Drizzle glaze over each scone. Sprinkle each with crushed pepitas.

19. Gingerbread Cut-Out Cookies

Prep Time: 20 mins

Cook Time: 10 mins

Total Time: 30 mins

Yield: 24 Cookies

Ingredients

- 1 ½ cups all-purpose flour

- 1 cup whole wheat pastry flour

- ¾ tablespoon ground cinnamon

- ½ tablespoon ground ginger

- ¼ teaspoon ground cloves

- ½ teaspoon baking soda

- ½ teaspoon coarse salt

- ½ cup softened butter

- ½ cup dark brown sugar

- ½ cup molasses

- 1 large egg

- 3–4 tablespoons milk

- Flour, for dusting

- ¼ cup powdered sugar and/or white icing

Instructions

1. Preheat oven to 350 degrees. Line a large cookie sheet with parchment paper.

2.In a large mixing bowl, whisk together flours, cinnamon, ginger, cloves, baking soda and salt until combined.

3.In a separate bowl, use a hand mixer to beat together softened butter and brown sugar until fluffy. Beat in egg and molasses, milk. Pour wet ingredients into the bowl with dry ingredients and use a spatula to mix together until combined and a dough ball has formed.

4.Dust a few tablespoons of flour on a large cutting board. Place dough on the cutting board and use a rolling pin to roll it out flat to about ¼ inch thickness. Use a gingerbread man cookie cutter and cut out about 24 cookies. Place them on the parchment paper, about ½ an inch apart. Bake 8-9 minutes, until set but soft.

5.Let cookies cool, then dust with powdered sugar or decorate with white icing.

20. Cranberry Pecan Pie Bars

Prep Time: 10 mins

Cook Time: 45 mins

Total Time: 55 mins

Yield: 12 Bars

Ingredients

Crust:

- 5 tablespoons cold butter, cubed
- ¾ cup Bob's Red Mill All-Purpose Organic Flour
- ¼ cup old-fashioned rolled oats
- 2 tablespoons ground flax seed
- 3 tablespoons maple syrup

Filling:

- 1 cup whole cranberries
- 1 cup chopped pecans
- ¼ cup granulated sugar
- 3 tablespoons maple syrup
- 1 tablespoon corn starch
- 1 ½ tablespoons melted butter
- ¼ teaspoon coarse salt

Instructions

1. Preheat oven to 350 degrees. Line an 8×8 baking dish with parchment paper and set aside.

2. Place crust ingredients into the bowl of a food processor and pulse until a crumbly dough forms. Press into the prepared baking dish until flat and even and bake 25 minutes, until slightly browned and set. Let crust slightly cool.

3. In a medium mixing bowl, stir together filling ingredients until combined. Pour filling onto the crust and bake an additional 15-20 minutes, until filling is set. Refrigerate until bars are completely cooled, then remove from the pan by pulling the parchment paper out onto a flat surface. Slice into bars and serve.

21. Italian Sausage & Tortellini Soup

Prep Time: 5-10 mins

Cook Time: 10-15 mins

Total Time: 15-25 mins

Yield: Serves 8

Ingredients

- 1 tablespoon olive oil
- 1-pound ground hot or mild Italian sausage
- 2 cloves garlic, peeled and minced
- 4–5 cups baby spinach
- 15-ounce can cannellini beans, drained and rinsed
- 2 teaspoons dried oregano leaves
- ½ teaspoon coarse salt
- ½ teaspoon freshly ground black pepper
- 2 (32-ounce) containers unsalted chicken stock
- 12-ounce bag fresh cheese tortellini
- Freshly shaved Parmesan cheese, for garnish

Instructions

1. Heat oil in a large Dutch oven or stock pot to
   medium heat. Add sausage and cook 4-5 minutes,
   until browned, breaking it up with a wooden spoon
   as it cooks.

2. Stir in the garlic and spinach and saute until
   spinach is wilted, about 2 minutes. Add cannellini
   beans, oregano, salt and pepper.

3. Add the stock to pot and bring to a simmer. Add
   tortellini and reduce heat to medium and allow to
   simmer, about 7-8 minutes, until tortellini is
   cooked. Taste and adjust seasoning, if necessary.

4. Serve in bowls and garnish with Parmesan cheese.

22. Sheet Pan Sausage & Potatoes

Prep Time: 5-10 mins

Cook Time: 25-35 mins

Total Time: 30-45 mins

Yield: Serves 4

Ingredients

- 12 ounces smoked sausage, sliced into rounds
- 1 ½ pounds baby red or Yukon potatoes, cubed
- 2 bell peppers, cored, seeded and sliced
- 2 tablespoons olive oil
- 1 ½ tablespoons Italian seasoning
- 1 teaspoon coarse salt
- ½ teaspoon ground black pepper
- ¼ teaspoon crushed red pepper flakes

Instructions

1. Preheat the oven to 400 degrees.

2. Coat a large baking sheet with cooking spray. Arrange the sausage, potatoes and bell peppers on the baking sheet and drizzle with olive oil. Sprinkle with Italian

seasoning, salt, black pepper and red pepper flakes. Toss to coat.

3. Roast 25-35 minutes, stirring halfway, or until potatoes are fork tender and sausage, potatoes and bell peppers and lightly browned. Serve.

23. Carrot Fries with Chipotle Aioli

Prep Time: 10-15 mins

Cook Time: 15-20 mins

Total Time: 25-35 mins

Yield: Serves 6

Ingredients

Chipotle Aioli:

- 6 ounces plain Greek yogurt
- 2 tablespoons mayonnaise
- 2 chipotle chilies, finely chopped + 2 tablespoons adobo sauce
- Zest and juice of 1 lime
- 2 teaspoons chili powder
- 1 teaspoon honey
- Dash coarse salt and ground black pepper

Carrot Fries:

- 2 pounds carrots, cut into fry shape
- 1 tablespoon oil

- Dash coarse salt and ground black pepper
- 2 tablespoons fresh cilantro, chopped (optional)

Instructions

1. Preheat grill to medium-high heat or oven to 425 degrees.

2. To make aioli, whisk together yogurt, mayonnaise, chilies with adobo sauce, lime zest and juice, chili powder and honey. Season with salt and pepper; stir to combine. Taste and adjust seasoning, if necessary. Refrigerate until ready to use.

3. Drizzle carrots with oil and season with salt and pepper. Toss to coat. Place carrot fries on preheated grill against the grates, cooking for 15-20 minutes, turning regularly. Or, if you're making them in the oven, line on a baking sheet and roast 15-20 minutes. Remove carrot fries and drizzle with chipotle aioli and garnish with chopped cilantro.

24. Cheesy Taco Pasta

Prep Time: 10-15 mins

Cook Time: 20-25 mins

Total Time: 30-40 mins

Yield: Serves 8

Ingredients

- 1-pound whole grain macaroni or shells
- 1 tablespoon oil
- ½ medium yellow onion, peeled and diced
- 1-pound lean ground beef, turkey or chicken
- 3–4 cloves garlic, peeled and minced
- 2 ½ tablespoons chili powder
- 1 tablespoon ground cumin
- 2 teaspoons smoked paprika
- 1 ¾ teaspoons coarse salt
- ½ teaspoon ground black pepper
- 15-ounce can black beans, rinsed and drained
- 15-ounce can fire roasted diced tomatoes
- ½ cup unsalted chicken, vegetable or beef stock
- ½ cup evaporated milk
- 1 ½ cups shredded cheddar cheese

- ½ cup fresh cilantro leaves, chopped

- Diced avocado, sour cream and crushed tortilla chips, for serving

Instructions

1. Bring a large pot of water to a boil. Cook pasta according to package directions. Drain and set aside.

2. In a large skillet or Dutch oven, heat oil to medium. Add the onion and sauté 3-4 minutes or until slightly soft. Add the ground beef and cook 7-8 minutes or until the beef is browned, breaking it up with a wooden spoon as it cooked. Stir in the garlic, chili powder, cumin, smoked paprika, salt and black pepper and sauté 30-60 seconds or until fragrant.

3. Add the black beans, tomatoes, stock and evaporated milk to the pot and bring to a simmer. Remove from the heat and stir in the cheddar cheese until melted. Add the pasta and cilantro and stir to combine. Taste and adjust seasoning, if necessary.

4. Serve taco pasta in bowls topped with avocado, sour cream and crushed tortilla chips.

25. Tater Tot Casserole

Prep Time: 15-20 mins

Cook Time: 35-40 mins

Total Time: 50 mins – 1 hr

Yield: Serves 8

Ingredients

- 3 tablespoons oil or butter
- ½ medium onion, peeled and diced
- 1-pound lean ground beef
- 12-ounce bag frozen mixed vegetables
- 1 ½ teaspoons kosher or sea salt
- 1 teaspoon dried mustard powder
- ½ teaspoon each celery salt, onion powder and garlic powder
- ½ teaspoon ground black pepper
- 4 tablespoons all-purpose flour
- 2 cups unsalted beef stock
- Dash Worcestershire sauce (optional)
- ½ cup shredded cheddar cheese
- ~70-75 frozen tater tots (from a 32-ounce bag)

Instructions

1. Preheat the oven to 375 degrees.

2. Heat the oil or butter in a large stove-top casserole dish or large oven-safe skillet to medium. Add the onion and sauté 4-5 minutes or until soft. Add the ground beef and cook another 5-7 minutes or until browned, breaking up the pieces with a wooden spoon as it cooks. Stir in the mixed vegetables and sauté another 2-3 minutes. Stir in the salt, mustard powder, celery salt, onion powder, garlic powder and black pepper.

3. Stir in the flour until incorporated. Increase the heat to medium-high. Add the stock and bring to a simmer, stirring constantly for 2-3 minutes, until thickened. Taste and adjust the seasoning, if necessary. Stir in the Worcestershire sauce (if using). Remove from the heat and flatten the beef mixture in an even layer.

4. Sprinkle the cheddar cheese in an even layer over the beef mixture. Line with tater tots. Bake 20-25 minutes or until the tater tots are golden and crispy and the

filling is bubbly. Let rest for 5 minutes, then scoop
and serve.

Prep Time: 10 mins

Cook Time: 20 mins

Total Time: 30 mins

Yield: Serves 6

Ingredients

- 12-ounce box whole grain spaghetti
- ¼ cup + 1 tablespoon extra virgin olive oil
- 4 cloves garlic, minced
- 3 large egg yolks, beaten
- 1 cup cooked baby peas
- ½ cup freshly shaved Parmesan cheese, divided
- Coarse salt and freshly ground black pepper, to taste
- Fresh lemon zest and juice, to taste

Instructions

1. Bring a large pot of salted water to a boil. Cook pasta according to package directions, until al dente.

2. Drain pasta, reserving 1 ¼ cups pasta water for later use. Coat pasta with 1 Tbsp. olive oil and set aside.

3. Place ¼ cup olive oil in the large pot on medium-high heat. Add garlic and cook until fragrant, about 30-60 seconds. Add pasta back in to the stock pot, then the pasta water and simmer until liquid is reduced by half. Remove from the heat and stir in the beaten egg yolks until it starts to thicken.

4. Stir in peas and half the Parmesan cheese.

5. Season with salt, black pepper and lemon zest and juice, to taste. Remove from heat and place in bowls.

6. Garnish with remaining Parmesan cheese.

27. Creamy Chicken & Wild Rice Soup

Prep Time: 20 min

Cook Time: 45 min

Total Time: 1 hr 5 min

Yield: Serves 8

Ingredients

- 4 tablespoons butter or oil
- 1 medium yellow or white onion, peeled and diced
- 2 medium carrots, peeled and diced
- 1 medium stalk celery, diced
- 1 ½ pounds boneless skinless chicken breasts, diced
- 2–3 cloves garlic, peeled and minced
- 2 teaspoons poultry seasoning
- 1–1 ½ teaspoons coarse salt
- 1 teaspoon dried mustard powder
- 1 teaspoon celery salt
- ¾ teaspoon ground black pepper
- 4 tablespoons all-purpose flour
- 5–6 cups unsalted chicken stock*
- 1 cup wild rice or wild rice blend

- 2–3 sprigs fresh thyme

- 2 dried bay leaves

- 3–4 tablespoons heavy cream or half and half

- 1 teaspoon Worcestershire sauce or low sodium soy sauce (optional)

Instructions

1. In a Dutch oven or stock pot, heat olive oil to medium. Add onion, carrots and celery and cook 7-8 minutes or until soft.

2. Add the diced chicken breast and cook until slightly browned on the outside.

3. Stir in garlic, poultry seasoning, salt, mustard powder, celery salt and black pepper. Stir in flour.

4. Add chicken stock and turn heat to medium-high. Bring to a simmer, then add wild rice, thyme sprigs and bay leaves. Reduce heat to low and let simmer, stirring frequently, for 40-50 minutes or until rice is al dente, adding additional stock if mixture gets too thick or starts to stick to the bottom.

5. Remove the thyme sprigs and bay leaves and discard. Stir in cream or half and half. Add Worcestershire or soy sauce, if desired. Taste and adjust seasoning, if necessary.

Prep Time: 20 mins

Cook Time: 35 mins

Total Time: 55 mins

Yield: 8 servings

Ingredients

Stew:

- 4 tablespoons butter or oil
- 2 pounds boneless skinless chicken breasts or thighs*
- 1–1 ½ teaspoons coarse salt, divided
- ½ teaspoon ground black pepper, divided
- 1 medium yellow onion, peeled and diced
- 3–4 carrots, peeled and chopped
- 3–4 stalks celery, chopped
- 4 tablespoons all-purpose flour
- 6 cups unsalted chicken stock
- 2 bay leaves
- 3–4 sprigs fresh thyme
- ¼ teaspoon celery salt

- ¼ teaspoon dried mustard powder
- 1 cube all-natural bouillon (optional)

Dumplings:

- 2 cups whole wheat pastry flour
- 1 tablespoon baking powder
- ½ teaspoon baking soda
- ½ teaspoon coarse salt
- 4 tablespoons melted butter
- 1 cup milk or buttermilk

Instructions

1. Heat butter or oil in a large Dutch oven to medium heat. Season chicken breasts or thighs with a pinch of the salt and pepper, then place in the hot butter or oil and cook 4-5 minutes per side. Remove from the pot and place on a cutting board. Shred or chop into bite-sized pieces.

2. Add onion, carrot and celery to the pot. Cook on medium, stirring occasionally, for 6-7 minutes, until soft. Stir in flour, increase heat to medium-high, then whisk in chicken stock. Add chicken back to the pot. Add bay leaves and thyme sprigs to the stock. Bring to

a simmer, stirring occasionally, until thickened, about 4-5 minutes. Whisk in remaining salt, pepper, celery salt, mustard powder and bouillon, if using. Taste and adjust seasonings, if necessary. Reduce heat to medium and remove discard the bay leaves and thyme sprigs.

3. In a medium mixing bowl, stir together flour, baking powder, baking soda, and salt. Stir in butter and milk until combined. Drop 8 balls of dough into the pot. Cook for 12-15 minutes with the lid on, until dumplings are soft and cooked through.

29. Carrot Fries with Chipotle Aioli

Prep Time: 10-15 mins

Cook Time: 15-20 mins

Total Time: 25-35 mins

Yield: Serves 6

Ingredients

Chipotle Aioli:

- 6 ounces plain Greek yogurt
- 2 tablespoons mayonnaise
- 2 chipotle chilies, finely chopped + 2 tablespoons adobo sauce
- Zest and juice of 1 lime
- 2 teaspoons chili powder
- 1 teaspoon honey
- Dash coarse salt and ground black pepper

Carrot Fries:

- 2 pounds carrots, cut into fry shape
- 1 tablespoon oil
- Dash coarse salt and ground black pepper
- 2 tablespoons fresh cilantro, chopped (optional)

Instructions

1. Preheat grill to medium-high heat or oven to 425 degrees.

2. To make aioli, whisk together yogurt, mayonnaise, chilies with adobo sauce, lime zest and juice, chili powder and honey. Season with salt and pepper; stir to combine. Taste and adjust seasoning, if necessary. Refrigerate until ready to use.

3. Drizzle carrots with oil and season with salt and pepper. Toss to coat. Place carrot fries on preheated grill against the grates, cooking for 15-20 minutes, turning regularly. Or, if you're making them in the oven, line on a baking sheet and roast 15-20 minutes. Remove carrot fries and drizzle with chipotle aioli and garnish with chopped cilantro.

Prep Time: 10-15 mins

Cook Time: 15-20 mins

Total Time: 25-35 mins

Yield: Serves 6

Ingredients

- 1-pound whole grain gnocchi
- 2 tablespoons olive oil
- ½ medium yellow onion, peeled and diced
- 1 medium red bell pepper, stemmed and diced
- 4 ears sweet corn, cut from the cob
- 2 medium zucchinis, diced
- 4 cloves garlic, peeled and minced
- 3 tablespoons half and half
- Zest and juice of 1 medium lime (about 2 tablespoons)
- 1 ¼ teaspoons kosher or sea salt
- ½ teaspoon ground black pepper
- ½ cup freshly grated Parmesan cheese, divided
- ½ cup fresh basil leaves, chiffonade

Instructions

1. Bring a large stock pot of water to a boil. Add the gnocchi and cook 4-5 minutes or until the gnocchi float to the surface. Drain and set aside.

2. Heat the olive oil in a large skillet to medium. Add the onion, bell pepper and sweet corn and sauté 4-5 minutes or until soft. Stir in the gnocchi, zucchini and garlic and sauté 1-2 minutes or until gnocchi is lightly browned. Stir in the half and half, lime zest and juice, salt, black pepper, and half of the Parmesan cheese. Bring to a simmer for 2-3 minutes. Stir in half of the basil.

3. Serve gnocchi skillet in bowls and top with remaining Parmesan cheese and basil.

31. Antipasto Ham Roll-Ups

Prep Time: 10-15 mins

Total Time: 10-15 mins

Yield: Makes 10 roll ups

Ingredients

- ½ pound deli ham slices
- 10 slices mozzarella or provolone cheese
- 2 ounces cream cheese, softened
- Freshly ground black pepper and crushed red pepper flakes
- ½ cup chopped sun-dried tomatoes
- ½ cup sliced black olives
- ½ cup marinated artichoke hearts, chopped
- Small handful fresh oregano leaves

Instructions

1. Lay 10 slices of deli ham on a cutting board. Top each with a slice of mozzarella or provolone cheese, then smear with a thin layer of cream cheese, all the way out to the edges. Sprinkle with a pinch of black pepper

and red pepper flakes. Top each with a few sun-dried tomatoes, black olives and artichoke hearts, then sprinkle with fresh oregano leaves.

2. Gently roll, tucking the filling in as you go. If roll-up doesn't stay secured, add a dab of cream cheese under the edge to help hold it together. Repeat with remaining roll-ups.

32. Sweet Potato Skin Chips

Prep Time: 10 mins

Cook Time: 30 mins

Total Time: 40 mins

Yield: 4 Servings

Ingredients

- 4–5 medium sweet potatoes, washed
- 1 tablespoon olive or grapeseed oil
- Pinch coarse salt
- Pure maple syrup, for drizzling (optional)
- Pinch dried rosemary, for garnish (optional)

Instructions

1. Preheat oven to 400 degrees.

2. Peel sweet potatoes using a chef's knife, creating large skins with just a little flesh attached. (Set aside sweet potato flesh for another use.)

3. Place sweet potato skins on a baking sheet and toss with oil and a pinch of salt. Bake for 25-30 minutes, until skins and crispy and brown. Allow to cool.

4. Drizzle with maple syrup and sprinkle with dried rosemary, if using. Serve.

33. Broccoli Cheddar Bites

Prep Time: 10-15 mins

Cook Time: 15-20 mins

Total Time: 25-35 mins

Yield: 18 broccoli bites

Ingredients

- 4 cups cooked broccoli florets
- 2–3 slices cooked bacon
- 2 large eggs
- ¾ cup shredded sharp or mild cheddar cheese
- 2 tablespoons + ¼ cup panko breadcrumbs, divided
- ½ teaspoon garlic powder
- ½ teaspoon onion powder
- ½ teaspoon coarse salt
- ¼ teaspoon ground black pepper
- Pinch crushed red pepper flakes (optional)

Instructions

1. Place broccoli and bacon in a food processor*. Pulse until broccoli and bacon are in small crumbles. Place broccoli/bacon crumbles in a medium bowl. Add eggs,

cheese, 2 tablespoons breadcrumbs, garlic powder, onion powder, salt, black pepper and red pepper flakes, if using. Stir to combine. Place mixture in the freezer for 1 hour or refrigerator for at least 2 hours, until chilled.

2. Preheat oven to 400 degrees. Coat a baking sheet with cooking spray and set aside.

3. Using a medium cookie scoop, form balls of mixture, using hands to shape. Roll in remaining ¼ cup breadcrumbs until coated. Place on baking sheet, about ½ inch apart. Coat bites with cooking spray. Bake 15-20 minutes, until breadcrumbs are crispy and lightly browned. Allow to cool slightly before eating.

Prep Time: 10-15 mins

Cook Time: 15-20 mins

Total Time: 25-35 mins

Yield: Makes 18 meatballs

Ingredients

Chicken Meatballs:

- 1 ¼ pounds ground chicken breast
- 2 cups fresh spinach, finely chopped
- 6-ounces crumbled feta cheese
- ½ cup panko bread crumbs
- 1 large egg
- 1 ½ tablespoons Dijon or horseradish mustard
- 1 tablespoon minced onion
- 1 teaspoon dried oregano leaves
- 1 teaspoon dried dill leaves
- ¾ teaspoon coarse salt
- ¼ teaspoon ground black pepper

Dill Pesto:

- 3 cups fresh spinach

- ¼ cup fresh baby dill

- 2 cloves garlic, peeled

- 3 tablespoons pine nuts (or other nut)

- Zest and juice of ¼ lemon

- ½ teaspoon coarse salt

- ¼ teaspoon ground black pepper

- ⅓ cup olive oil

Instructions

1. Preheat oven to 375 degrees. Prepare a baking sheet fitted with a wire rack and coat with cooking spray. Set aside.

2. In a large bowl, thoroughly mix together all of the meatball ingredients. Using your hands, form 2-inch meatballs and place on the wire rack with an inch of space in between meatballs.

3. Bake for 10-12 minutes, until internal temperature of meatballs reach 160 degrees.

4. While meatballs cook, place spinach, dill, garlic, pine nuts, lemon juice and a pinch of salt and pepper in the bowl of a food processor. Process while drizzling olive

oil in through the vegetable shoot, until desired consistency is reached. Taste and adjust seasoning, if necessary.

35. Crock Pot Apple Fritter Bread

Prep Time: 15 mins

Cook Time: 2 hrs

Total Time: 2 hrs 15 mins

Yield: Serves 12

Ingredients

- 0.25-ounce package active dry yeast (about 2 ¼ teaspoons)
- 1 tablespoon honey
- 1 ¼ cups warm water
- 1 ½ teaspoons coarse salt
- 3 cups whole wheat pastry flour + a few spoonfuls
- 2 tablespoons ground flax seed (optional)
- 3 medium sweet apples, diced
- ½ cup walnuts, chopped
- 2 tablespoons butter, melted
- 1 ½ teaspoons cinnamon
- 2 tablespoons brown sugar

Instructions

1. Place yeast, honey and warm water in the bowl of a stand mixer. Whisk to combine. Allow to sit for 15-20 minutes, until mixture has puffed up.

2. Fit mixer with dough hook. Stir in salt, then mix in flour, ½ cup at a time, with the mixer running on low. Mix in flax seed, if using. Allow dough to mix on low for 4-5 minutes, until a ball has formed. Dough should be slightly sticky. Mix in diced apple and walnuts until combined.

3. Place a few spoonfuls of flour on a large piece of parchment paper. Transfer dough to the paper and form a ball. Place a damp cloth over the dough and allow to rise for about 1 hour or until dough has doubled in size. Transfer dough with the parchment paper into the crock pot. Set on low.

4. Whisk together melted butter, cinnamon and brown sugar in a liquid measuring cup. Pour mixture over dough and swirl it into the dough with a butter knife. Place the lid on the crock pot and allow to cook for 1 to

2 hours, until internal temperature of bread reaches 190-200 degrees.

36. Thanksgiving Leftovers Gravy Balls

Prep Time: 10-15 mins

Cook Time: 20-25 mins

Total Time: 30-40 mins

Yield: Makes 16 balls

Ingredients

- 2 cups cooked turkey, coarsely chopped
- 1 ½ cups leftover stuffing
- 1 ½ cups leftover mashed potatoes
- 1 large egg
- 2 tablespoons milk
- ½ cup panko breadcrumbs
- ½ cup leftover gravy and/or cranberry sauce

Instructions

1. Preheat oven to 375 degrees.

2. Fit baking sheet with a wire rack and coat with cooking spray. Set aside.

3. Mix together chopped turkey, stuffing and mashed potatoes in a bowl until thoroughly combined, like

meatloaf. Using your hands, roll mixture into about 16 medium-sized balls.

4. In a small bowl, whisk together egg and milk. Place breadcrumbs in a medium-sized bowl. Coat each ball with egg wash, then breadcrumbs and place on the wire rack. Coat balls with cooking spray. Bake for 15 minutes, until outside is crispy.

5. Turn oven to a low broil and toast balls for about 4 minutes, turning occasionally so all sides are evenly browned.

6. Serve with reheated gravy or cranberry sauce.

Prep Time: 1 hr

Cook Time: 40 mins

Total Time: 1 hr 40 mins

Yield: 12 Bars

Ingredients

- 1 ¼ cups white whole wheat, oat or almond flour
- 1 ¼ cups old fashioned rolled oats
- ½ teaspoon coarse salt
- ½ teaspoon baking soda
- ½ cup honey
- ½ cup packed light-brown sugar
- 4 tablespoons butter, melted
- 1 teaspoon vanilla extract
- Ice cold water (optional)
- ½ cup fat free sweetened condensed milk
- ½ cup low fat evaporated milk
- 15-ounce can pumpkin puree
- 2 large eggs
- 1 teaspoon pumpkin pie spice

Instructions

1. Preheat oven to 350°F. In a medium mixing bowl, whisk together flour, oats, salt and baking soda. Stir in honey and brown sugar and mix until no clumps remain. Stir vanilla into melted butter and pour mixture over dry ingredients. Using a spoon, stir mixture until evenly moistened. If it is too dry, add 1 tablespoon of ice water at a time until it has a formed consistency. Sprinkle half of the crumb mixture into the bottom of a greased 8×8 baking dish and gently press into an even layer. Bake in preheated oven for 15 minutes. Remove from the oven and set aside.

2. In a mixing bowl, whisk together milks, pumpkin, eggs and pumpkin pie spice until well blended. Pour mixture over crumb crust in baking dish and spread into an even layer. Sprinkle top evenly with remaining crumb mixture. Bake in preheated oven 25-30 minutes, until lightly golden. Remove from the oven and allow to cool at room temperature. Once cool, cover and refrigerate 30 minutes to 1 hour, then remove and cut into squares. Store in airtight container in the refrigerator.

39. Chicken Taco Casserole

Prep Time: 10-15 mins

Cook Time: 20-25 mins

Total Time: 30-40 mins

Yield: Serves 10

Ingredients

- 1 tablespoon olive oil
- 3 tablespoons taco seasoning, divided (see recipe in notes)
- 1-pound boneless skinless chicken breasts
- 2 cups cooked brown rice
- 15-ounce can pinto beans, drained and rinsed
- ½ cup canned or frozen mexi-corn
- 2 bell peppers, seeded and sliced or diced
- 2 (10-ounce) cans diced tomatoes with green chilies, drained
- 4-ounce can diced green chilies
- 4-ounce can diced jalapenos (optional)
- 10-ounce can salsa verde
- Dash coarse salt and ground black pepper*
- 1 ½ cups shredded sharp cheddar cheese, divided

- ½ cup shredded pepper jack cheese, divided
- ½ bag tortilla chips
- Cilantro, green onion, avocado, plain Greek yogurt for garnish

Instructions

1. Preheat oven to 375 degrees.

2. Heat olive oil in a skillet to medium heat. Season chicken breasts with 1 tablespoon taco seasoning. Place chicken in the hot skillet and saute 3-5 minutes on each side, until chicken is browned and juices run clear. Remove from the pan and allow to rest 5-10 minutes. Chop chicken into small pieces.

3. In a large bowl, combine chicken pieces, brown rice, pinto beans, corn, bell peppers, tomatoes, green chilies, jalapenos (if using), salsa verde, remaining taco seasoning, salt and pepper.

4. Place mixture into a greased baking dish and top with half of both cheeses. Line the top with the tortilla chips and remaining cheeses. Bake for 15-20 minutes, until cheese is melted and bubbly.

5. Top casserole with cilantro, green onion, avocado
   and/or Greek yogurt.

40. Corn Chip-Crusted Chicken Nuggets

Prep Time: 10-15 mins

Cook Time: 15-20 mins

Total Time: 25-35 mins

Yield: Serves 4

Ingredients

Avocado Dip:

- 1 ripe avocado, peeled
- Zest and juice of 2 medium limes
- ½ cup plain Greek yogurt
- ¼ cup cilantro, chopped
- Pinch coarse salt
- 2 teaspoons granulated sugar

Chicken Nuggets:

- 3 ½ cups corn chips
- 1 teaspoon chili powder
- ½ teaspoon ground cumin
- ½ teaspoon smoked paprika

- Dash crushed red pepper flakes or cayenne pepper
- 1 large egg
- ½ cup milk
- 1-pound boneless skinless chicken breasts, cubed
- Pinch coarse salt and ground black pepper

Instructions

1. Puree avocado, lime, Greek yogurt, cilantro and sugar. Taste and adjust seasoning, if necessary. Place in the refrigerator.
2. Preheat oven to 375 degrees.
3. Combine the corn chips, chili powder, cumin, smoked paprika and red pepper flakes/cayenne in the bowl of a food processor. Pulse until mixture resembles bread crumbs. In a separate small bowl, whisk together egg and milk.

4. Season chicken breast cubes with a dash of salt and pepper. Prepare baking sheet with a wire rack and coat with cooking spray. Dip chicken breast cubes into the egg/milk mixture, then coat with the corn chip/spice mixture. Place on the wire rack with at least an inch of space in between each nugget. Coat each nugget with cooking spray. Place in the oven and

bake for 12-14 minutes, until internal temperature of nuggets reaches 160 degrees.

5. Allow nuggets to cool for a few minutes before eating. Serve with avocado yogurt dip.